SELFNESS

Simple Self-Care Secrets for Those Who Care for Others!

by

Carol L Rickard, LCSW, TTS

Has Appeared::

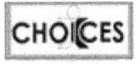
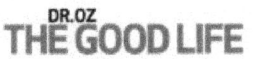

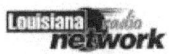
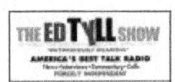
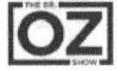
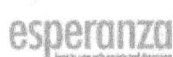
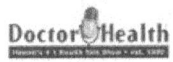

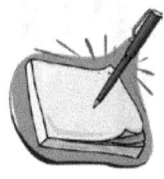

Sign up now!

To get access to updates, more tools, coaching calls, and upcoming events
Text: SELFNESS
To: **44222**

Copyright © 2017 Carol L Rickard

All rights reserved.

ISBN: 0-9908476-8-3
ISBN-13: 978-0-9908476-8-7

SELFNESS:
Simple Self-Care Secrets for Those Who Care for Others!

by Carol L Rickard, LCSW, TTS

All rights reserved. No part of this book may be reproduced for resale, redistribution, or any other purposes (including but not limited to eBooks, pamphlets, articles, video or audiotapes, & handouts or slides for lectures or workshops). Permission to reproduce these materials for those and any other purposes must be obtained in writing from the author.

The author & publisher of this book do not dispense medical advice nor prescribe the use of this material as a form of treatment. The author & publisher are not engaged in rendering psychological, medical, or other professional services.

The purpose of this material is educational only. Please see you doctor concerning any medical advice you may need.

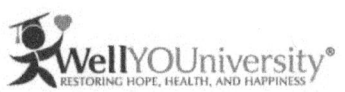

888 LIFE TOOLS (543-3866)

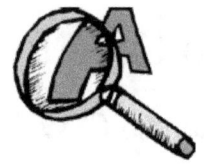

What will you get out of this book?

- A new way of looking at self-care!

- Increased awareness of WHY you need to *practice self-care!*

- Simple tools for getting the job done!

- Improved quality of life:
  your health, your relationship, your work!

Contents

About this book	1
Why I Wrote This Book	4
A Quick Check-in	6

Part I   A New Approach!

What is SELFNESS?	10
Getting Started	16

Part II   3 Keys to Self-Care Success

Key # 1 Use The Right Tools	33
Key # 2 Manage Your Emotions	47
Key # 3 Have a Solid Foundation	85
Wrapping Things Up	109
A Quick Check-out	115
Feedback Card	116
About the Author	117
Having Carol Speak	118
Well YOUniversity	119

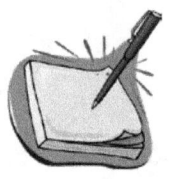

Sign up now!

To get access to updates, more tools, coaching calls, and upcoming events
Text: SELFNESS
To: **44222**

About This Book

In all my years of helping people successfully change health habits, **I've discovered:**

People are *already smart enough* when it comes to being healthy.

YOU KNOW *WHAT* TO DO!

It's the '*DOING*' or *lack of it* that keeps you stuck where you are.

I can help *change* that!

I doubt you have ever read a 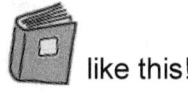 like this!

Unless, of course, you may have read any of my **8** other books.

* I like to think of my books as a workshop - only in print!*

Along with **simple** & easy to understand chapters, I tend to use a lot of pictures,

analogies

& word art

to make the information stick in the brain!

I like call my approach:

SMARTheory™

It's what makes my books and services *different* from all others!

KNOWLEDGE is the left brain at work.

This is where YOU *know* what to do!

Because I use "pictures" & "images", I end up *tapping in to the other side of the brain –*

the right side!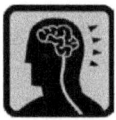

This is also the side that synthesizes things, like the operating system in a computer!

With both sides working on the 'same page',
the end result is getting people to

Move knowledge in to ACTION!

This book will introduce you to

my proven secrets for putting some

SELF-CARE in to your life

These are the ***very same things***

I have used myself for the past 25 years.

I am excited to be able to share them with you!

WHY I Wrote This Book!

This past year I was hired by RUTGERS

to create & lead a custom workshop on

self-care

for The Children's Home Society of New Jersey.

Okay, I'll admit.......

I was a little nervous when the day finally

came since it was all 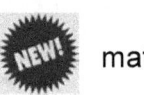 material.....

The ❓ 's whirled in my mind:

Would they:

    Stay engaged?

        Be interested?

            Walk away with the "tools"?

                Practice self-care more?

When we got to the end of the workshop, 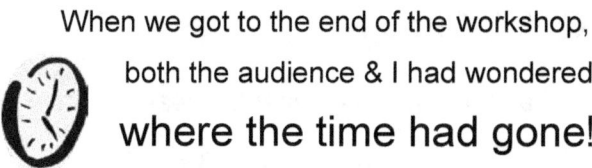 both the audience & I had wondered where the time had gone!

I knew then this had turned out to be a **GREAT** workshop!

Their words confirmed this as they left, thanking me for *"a great workshop"*!

I did this workshop a few more times….

Each time the results were the same:

People were walking away with **new tools**

&

a new commitment to **start practicing self-care** on a daily basis!

I want to share this same information with YOU!
It's time for you ***to start caring*** for YOU!

A Quick Check-In!

Just as I do in my live events, I want to have you measure 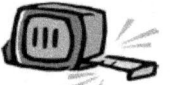 to see where you are starting from!

Circle the number below each statement that best describes where you are RIGHT NOW!

1) I feel I have enough self-care tools.

    0   1   2   3   4   5

not at all!   absolutely

2) I use self-care tools every day.

    0   1   2   3   4   5

not at all!   absolutely

3) I feel I have a right to take time for myself.

    0   1   2   3   4   5

not at all!   absolutely

Want a FREE 30 minute coaching call with me? Email me your scores when you're done reading!

I know this stuff works for me!

I want to be sure it works for YOU!

So at the end of the book,

You'll see the section: A Quick Check-Out!

Here you'll answer the same 3 questions again!

We'll be able to tell if this accomplishes what it is being written to do!

Give you more Self-Care Tools!

&

Get you practicing Self-Care daily!

See page 113 to see how you can get a FREE 30 minute Coaching call with me!
Limited to the first 100 people

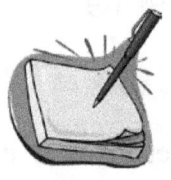

Sign up now!

To get access to updates, more tools, coaching calls, and upcoming events

Text: SELFNESS

To: **44222**

Part I
A New Approach!

What Is SELFNESS?

What Is SELFNESS?

Many years ago,
> I was running a therapy group
> with patients at the hospital.

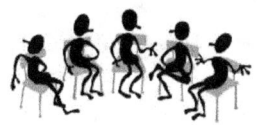

It was here that **SELFNESS** was born!

I had a patient I'll call Sue (not her real name!),
who was a single mom -

struggling & feeling overwhelmed.

I asked her to identify **1** thing
she could do for herself tonight.

Her response:

"I couldn't do anything for me."

 "I have to get the kids fed,
get them bathed & to bed,
& the laundry done."

I gently nudged her to think of something

she could 'do for herself'

that would *fit around those things.*

Her response:

"I couldn't – I've got too much to do."

I'd spent several years working

in a women's trauma program.

One of the self-care foundations we used was:

The Oxygen Mask!

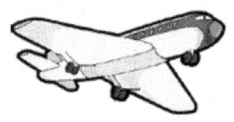

Since most people hadn't ever flown, I explained:

"When the oxygen masks drop from the ceiling &

you have a child or an adult who needs help –

Put the MASK ON YOURSELF first,

then help them."

Sue immediately stated:

"Oh I could never do that."
"I would put it on my children first."

To which I responded-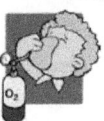

"Then you won't be around for the kids, *because* you'd pass out before you get yours on

& **they can't help you."**

Sue stuck to her answer: "I'd still do them first."

Huh? Her response didn't make sense to me so I asked why she wouldn't put it on herself first.

She said:

"That would be selfish."

I remember thinking

'Quick Carol, you've got to HELP her get this.'

Thank goodness my Higher Power helped & I quickly came up with my own reply:

"NO, that'd be practicing SELFNESS!
which is very different from selfish."

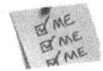

"*Selfish* is when we want other people to do what we want.

SELFNESS is when

we *take care of ourselves* 1ST

so we can be there to

take care of others who may be needing us!"

When I asked the group if this made sense?

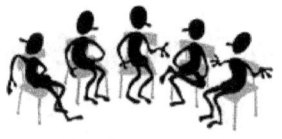

To my surprise, they all said yes, even Sue!
So I checked with her one last time....

"Sue, **who'd** you put the oxygen mask on *first*?"

She answered with a loud:

"MYSELF!"

And,

SELFNESS was born that day!

It doesn't get any **simpler than that!**

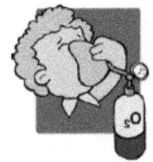

We MUST take care of ourselves
1ST

IF we want to be around

to take care of others!!!!

Join me in *making a commitment* to

PRACTICE SELFNESS EVERYDAY!

Getting Started!

At my live workshops,

the **1ST** thing I have people do is

take a bottle of A & W Root Beer

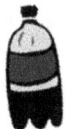 &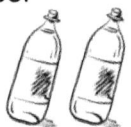

a large bottle of seltzer

and shake them up!

We pass the bottles around so we can get them *'really shook up!"*

If you feel brave & daring

so as to try this at home right now –

Go for it!

CAUTION!

Just make sure it is completely & tightly closed
BEFORE you start shaking and....

<u>DO NOT OPEN IT!</u>

Once you're done shaking it,

just set the bottle to the side.

** *Special Alert* **

One difference about doing this at 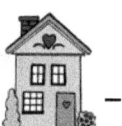 –

make sure you hide

the 'shook up' bottle

until you get to that part in the book!

You don't want anybody
else to find it &

accidently get a quick shower!

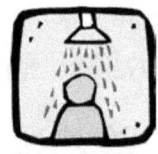

Let's move on to this:

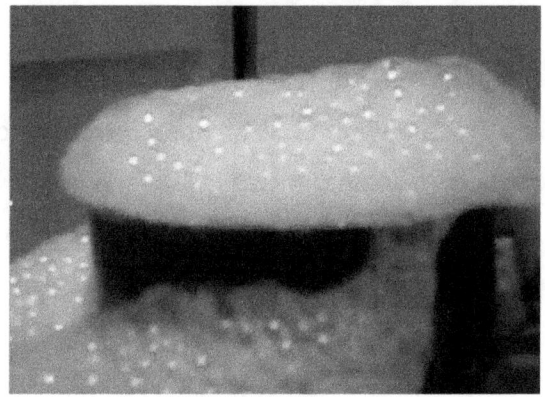

I call this:

THE SMART AUDIENCE TEST!

Raise your hand if you KNOW that once things get to this point you have a **real mess** to clean up!

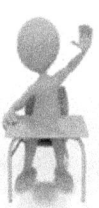

See, I knew you were SMART!

Well, the same principle applies to us!

When we *DON'T* practice self-care,

It too can lead to a real MESS!

Let's take a look:

What Mess?

What's *personal **mess*** of NOT practicing self-care?

Back in 2002, when I wasn't practicing self-care, here's the *personal **mess*** I was left to deal with:

MIGRAINES

OUT OF CONTROL

What is your PERSONAL *mess*?

Physical health? Emotional health?

Marriage or relationship? Unhealthy behaviors?

Take a moment & write down here **what happens TO YOU as the result of no self-care:**

When it comes to the PROFESSIONAL mess,

The most common result is

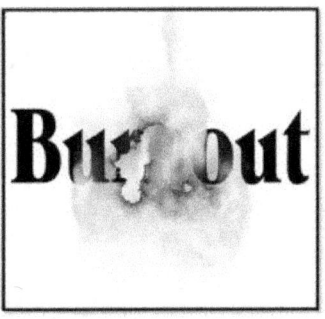

or

OVERLOAD!

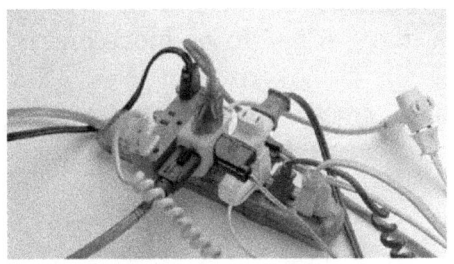

To *avoid both*

PERSONAL & PROFESSIONAL **messes**

There is ONLY

1 solution!!

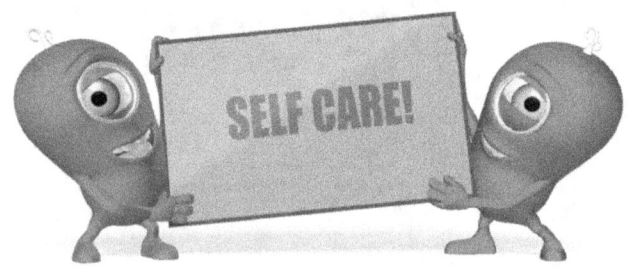

But WAIT! We still have a few more things

to cover *before* we move on to

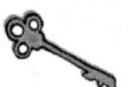

THE 3 KEYS TO

SELF-CARE SUCCESS!

Two birds are sitting on a wire.

One decides to fly away.

How many are left?

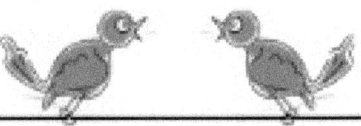

I like to start off my live workshops
with this little riddle.

It had such a tremendous impact on my life
the first time I heard it!

When they asked us to raise our hand
If we thought the answer was **one** -

My hand went up high & proud!
Wrong! The answer is two.

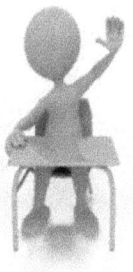

Oops!

DECIDING & DOING

are two different things!

Just because you decide to do something
DOESN'T mean that you DO it!

This was an Ah-Ha Moment for me -
There had been plenty of times
In my life when I **Decided**
&
I *NEVER* FOLLOWED THRU!

What about you?

Do you have times when you've *DECIDED*
& NOT followed through like me?

(This little riddle *helped me change that!*)

This is my wordtool to get moving!

Direct

Opportunity

© 2017 & licensed by Well YOUniversity, LLC
Taken from "Words at Work"

The same rule applies to this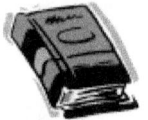

If you don't use what's in it,
it *won't work*.

KNOWING & DOING

are also two different things!

We either: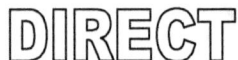

opportunity

or

IT gets *directed for us!*

And chances are it WON'T take us in
a direction of ***SELF-CARE!***

Is it worth the **COST**?

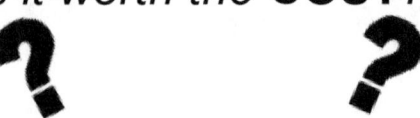

Here is what happens when we don't:

Denied

Opportunity

Not

'

Trying

© 2017 & licensed by Well YOUniversity, LLC
Taken from "Words at Work"

There are also many times when we *don't get to control the cards we are dealt.in life.*

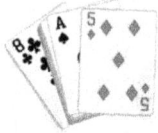

It's **in these times of challenge** when we need to be practicing SELF-CARE *even more!*

IT'S NOT

WHAT HAPPENS

TO YOU,

BUT

HOW YOU REACT

TO IT

THAT MATTERS

EPICTETUS

Or as Victor Frankl has pointed out:

> WHEN WE FACE A SITUATION
>
> THAT *CANNOT* BE CHANGED
>
> WE ARE **CHALLENGED**
> TO
> *CHANGE OURSELVES*
>
> VICTOR FRANKL

Please take a moment and write down below a few of the things you learned in this past chapter.

(Our brains hold on better to ideas when written!)

Part II

3 Keys to Self-Care Success!

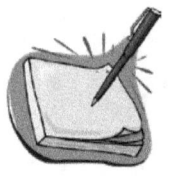

Sign up now!

To get access to updates, more tools, coaching calls, and upcoming events

Text: SELFNESS

To: **44222**

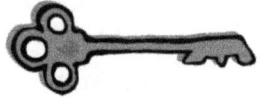

#1

Use the *Right Tools!*

I'm guessing you've a toolbox

or a drawer at home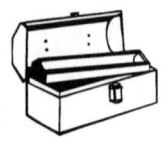

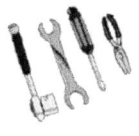 with some basic tools in it!

Just like we have

Tools for Things

we *need to have*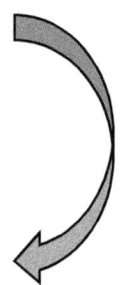

Tools for LIFE

I call them **LifeTOOLS**!

Now, let me ask you this question:

Have you ever taken one of these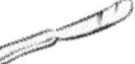

AND

Used it as one of these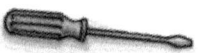

How'd that work for you?!

Now, *just in case* you're one of those people who answers:

"Not too bad."

I have one more question for you:

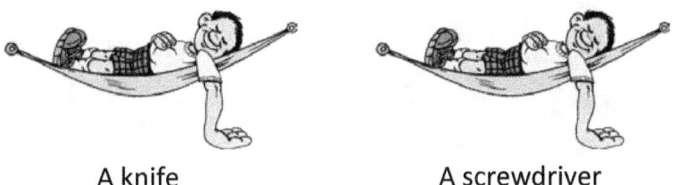

A knife   A screwdriver

I put together **2** hammocks,

ONE using a knife, ONE using a screwdriver.

Which one do you want to lay in?

The screwdriver, right?

The one using the knife will **MOST likely**

leave you on the ground after it **falls apart!**

What have you used

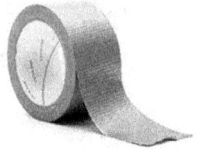

for?

Some of my uses have been:

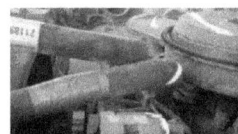

Radiator hose

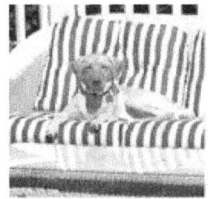

Lint brush

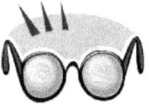

My Glasses

The knife & the duct tape are what I call:

Survival Tools

Things we grab at for a QUICK FIX!

Just like we have

Survival Tools for Things

We also have

Survival Tools for LIFE!

These are *the things* we grab at

when we get **stressed, angry, scared.....**

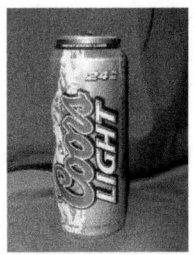

You are looking at one of my Survival Tools

The problem is -

I was only **14** at the time.

You see, I'd overheard a conversation right before
Christmas in 1976 & figured out
my father was going to die from cancer.

Now, I don't know about you....

but I grew up in a family

that really didn't talk about things.

So, I didn't tell anyone what I had overheard.

Instead, I started **stealing a lot**

of alcohol form my parents.

I remember taking a 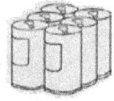 to school

in my blue Adidas bag,

putting it in my locker

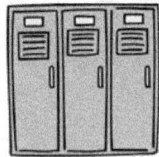

and then going out at lunch time to drink it.

If anyone had known

HOW MUCH I was drinking back then –

I am sure they would have had me in rehab!

I was very lucky though!

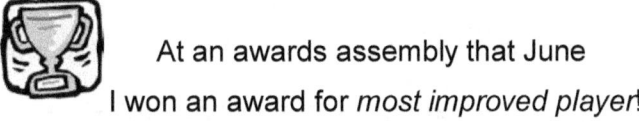 At an awards assembly that June
I won an award for *most improved player*!

It was a **life changing moment** for me....

I remember thinking: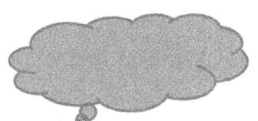

'Maybe I could be good at this.

Maybe I could use *this* to get to college.'

You see, my father had passed &

I'd already **started to *worry*** about

HOW I was going to be able to afford college.

So I *STOPPED* drinking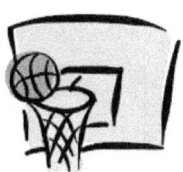

& focused all my time and energy on

Or as I like to say,

Basketball became my **LifeTOOL**!

I've found many people have things they USED to do when they were younger that served as their LifeTOOLS –

What about you?

Think back to when you were growing up –

What did you like or love to do?

It could be: sports, music, theatre, cheerleading, drawing, art, cars, cooking, being outdoors...

Just to name a few!

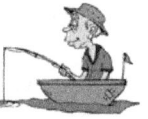

Take a moment to think back!

Whatever it was, write it in the box below:

There is one other example of Survival Tools
I'd like to share with you:

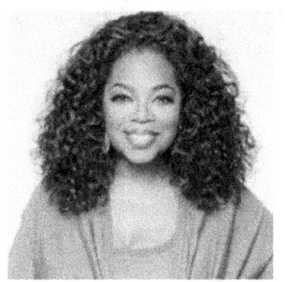

For many years,

Oprah battled with her weight.

SUCCESS *was* hers *once she realized*

FOOD was her **Survival Tool.**

The problem with Survival Tools:

They go on to become the problem!

It's like they take on a life of their own
that we are then *NOT ABLE* to manage.

Take a look at the following list

to see if you might have any

Survival Tools

Circle any of these that belong to you:

Eating / Food	Work
Shopping	Joking
Spending	Humor
Prescription Drug	Isolating
Smoking	Being quiet
Care*taking*	Independent
Risky Behavior	Don't trust
Fighting	Relationships
Avoiding	Being Angry
Worrying	Complaining
Sex	Self-Harm

Can you think of anymore???

A Key Point:

ANYTHING can become a Survival Tool

when it's used *to excess…..*

Or

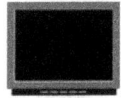 To **AVOID!**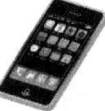

There's **1** other thing

I'd like to call your attention to –

If you look back at the list of

Survival Tools

you will see Care*taking* right in the middle.

This is written like this to get your attention!

Let me explain what this is:

Care*taking* = doing for someone WHO is ABLE to *take care of themselves!*

This is very different from CAREGIVING!

With Caregiving, we are doing for someone who is NOT ABLE to take care of themselves.

I have found people can get **so busy** *taking care of others* so they don't have to look at or deal with their own problems!

Need more tools?

Don't worry!

We'll get to many more LifeTOOLS

In the next chapter!!!!

If we are to be successful

Using the Right Tools,

Then we must get good at doing the following:

BECOME MORE **AWARE!**

Actively
Work
At
Recognizing
Existence

© 2017 & licensed by Well YOUniversity, LLC
Taken from "Words at Work"

We must become AWARE of

WHAT we are doing that *IS NOT* working

&

WHAT we are doing that **IS WORKING!**

After all,

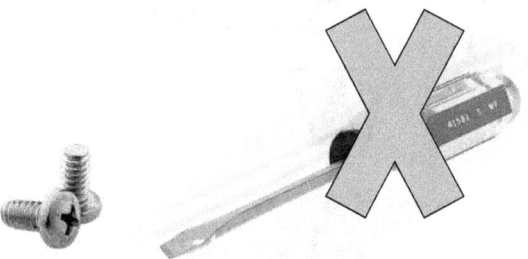

Using the RIGHT tool *makes* the difference

between **SUCCESS** & failure

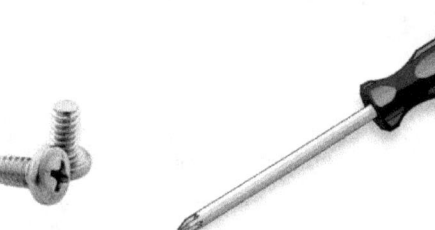

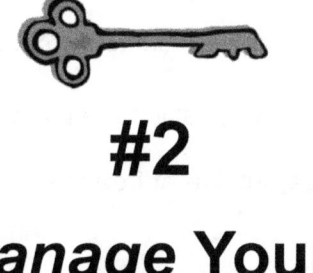

#2
Manage Your Emotions!

So let's move on to this next key:

Managing Your Emotions!

I have a few rules when it comes to this area I would like to go over 1st

They are critical to our **success**.

People don't usually have the chance to learn these outside of treatment programs.

So don't worry if you've never heard of them!

Carol's Rule #1

If we don't put words to feelings –

They come out as behaviors…

Carol's Rule #2

We have a right to our feelings,

We *don't* have a right to *take them out on others!*

Carol's Rule #3

Don't **BLAME!**

Here's what happens when we blame:

Become

Lost

Amongst

Many

Excuses!

© 2017 & licensed by Well YOUniversity, LLC
Taken from "Words at Work"

It only tends to make things

WORSE!

Now it's time to come back to the bottles
we *shook up* at the very beginning of the book!

Did you shake one up?

DON'T try to open it just yet...

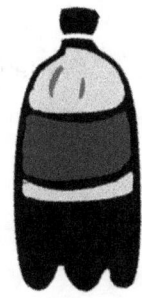

Why do I like to shake up a bottle?

Shake up a bottle
& PRESSURE builds up inside!

I think the same thing happens to us:

Life *SHAKES* us up
& FEELINGS builds up inside!

Maybe you've experienced this?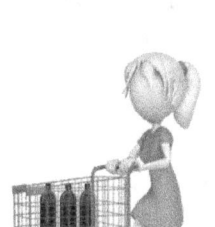
You go into a store & buy either a liter of
diet soda or some raspberry seltzer.

Along the way, you are very
careful not to shake it up!

That next week, you go to
pour yourself a glass, & not
paying attention you open it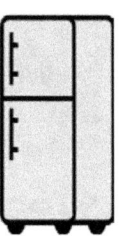

and …….

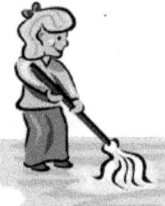

SPLASH…….

stuff comes flying out of the bottle you just opened -

all over you & the floor creating **a mess!**

I believe the same thing happens

When it comes to **our emotions!**

Sometimes **WE** get *shaken up!*

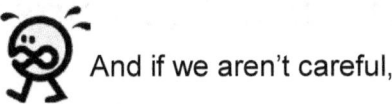 And if we aren't careful,

WE end up with a **BIG EMOTIONAL MESS!**

If we're to have any success with ***SELF-CARE***,

We must move away from using
SURVIVAL TOOLS

And start using *healthier ways* to manage our emotions!

Really, there are only 3 things we can do with our emotions……

"The Feelings Pendulum"

demonstrates this very nicely!

The Feelings Pendulum

What Do You Do With Your Feelings?

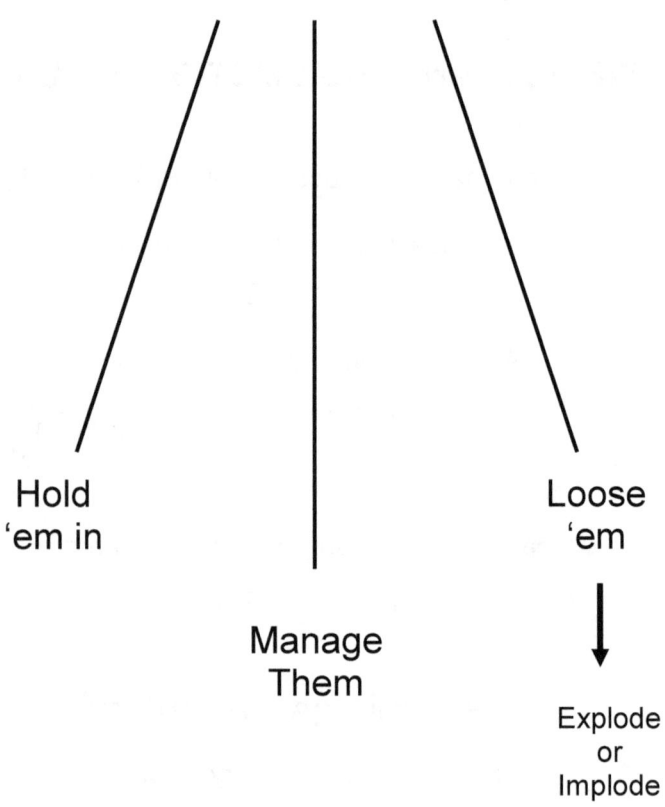

Let me explain what I mean by
EXPLODE & IMPLODE

Explode = emotions come out
& make a MESS!

Implode = emotions stay in &
you BECOME the MESS!

The BIG **?** is –

Where would you put yourself?

If it's '**MANAGE Them**' – *GREAT!*

If it's '**HOLD 'Em In**' – Don't worry!

If it's '**LOOSE 'Em**' – is that Explode
or Implode?

The KEY here is it can be difficult to

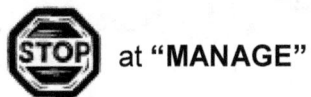 at **"MANAGE"**

When you start at either end!

Here's how our feelings & behaviors fit together:

It came to me when I was doing a group on anger.

I asked members what they did when angry.

Sue replied:

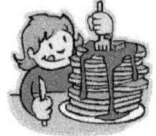 "I go to the kitchen & eat.
I can't help it."

What caught my attention was the

"I CAN'T HELP IT!"

You see, it might SEEM like we can't help it –

BUT we can!!!

And here's why"

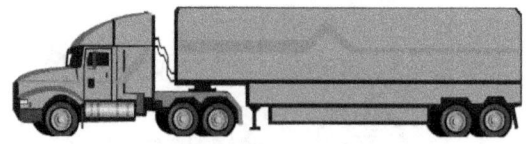

It seems to be one thing!

But is it?

When we take a closer look:

It's REALLY **2 parts!**

Just like our reactions have 2 parts!

FEELING   *BEHAVIOR:*

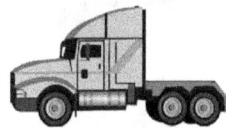 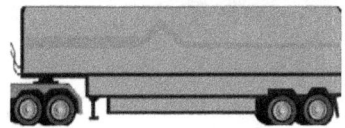

To Sue it feels like
her anger and her eating are 1 thing!

The truth is they *are not!*

When we experience situations in life
that *"shake up"* FEELINGS in us……

It is up to us to CHOOSE

what we will do with those FEELINGS!

We make the choice!

We decide which behavior we connect to!

Sue's ANGER

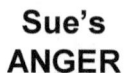
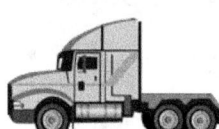
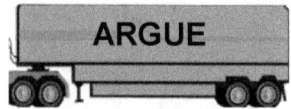
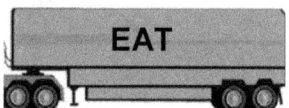
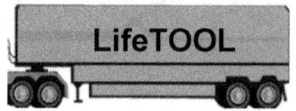

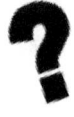 Which one will Sue CHOOSE!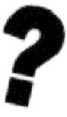

(Which one will *you* choose!)

For the **1000's** I have shared this idea with –

it becomes an   AH-HA Moment!

We are *responsible* for WHAT we DO with your feelings!

Here is the POWER of choice:

Controlling

How

Our

Intentions

Create

Experience

© 2017 & licensed by Well YOUniversity, LLC
Taken from "Words at Work"

YOU may need to make CHOICES

to avoid OVERLOAD!

Don't set yourself up to fail!

The Secret to **SUCCESS:**

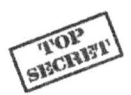

Choose a *new behavior*
you can *take action* on

Immediately!

Sadly,

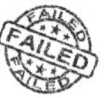

This is where I see most people......

get it WRONG!

They try to make *healthy changes* in their lives,
only to find themselves failing *miserably....*

Maybe this has happened to you in the past?

Again, it's one of those things I **only learned**
once I started working in treatment programs!

I love being able to share it with you!

Here's what I mean by this:

I asked Sue to pick one of the following *INSTEAD* of "eating" –

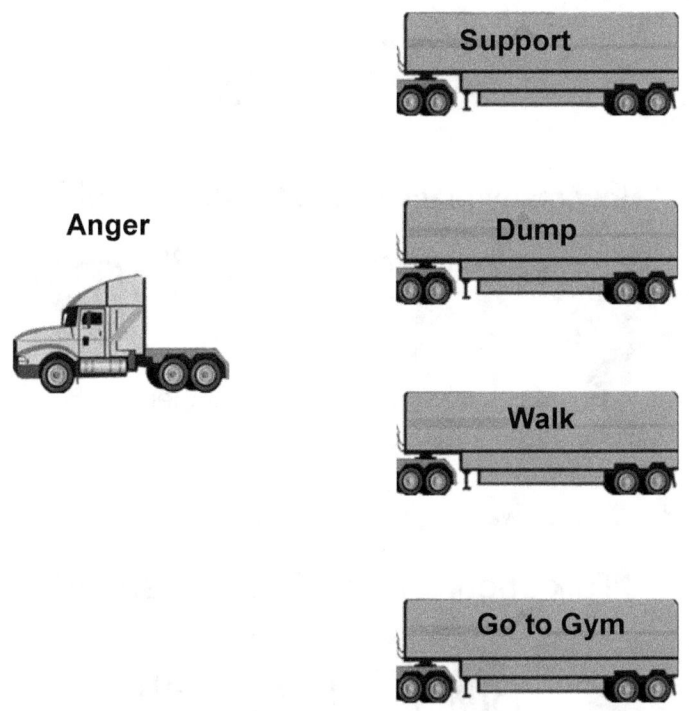

These are all healthy LifeTOOLS!

Her 1st pick was

"Go to Gym"

Then I asked:

"How long will it take to get to the gym?'

Sue replied, "It's a ½ hour from my house."

TOO LONG!!!!

How many places can she stop to EAT

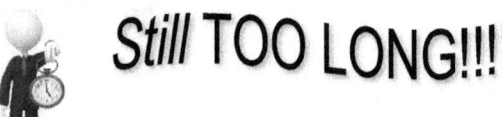

on the way to the gym?!

So I asked Sue to pick another!

Her 2nd pick was

"Talk about it in my Support Group"

 *Still* **TOO LONG!!!!**

WHY? It didn't meet until 3:00pm.

What happened if she got angry in the am?

So I hope you can see how Sue
was setting herself up to

She was picking other ✚ ways
to *manage her anger!*

The **problem** is they weren't
things she could take action on

Immediately!!

The remaining two choices were both things she
COULD DO right away:

Anger

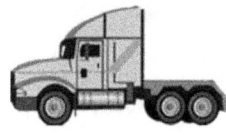

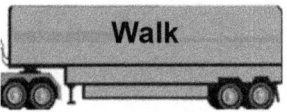

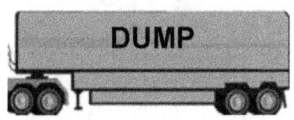

** I'll explain what ***DUMPING*** is in a minute!**

So it looks like one thing

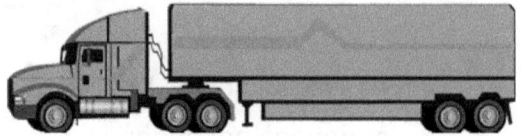

But it's important to remember –

IT'S NOT!!

FEELINGS & BEHAVIORS

Are 2 *Different*

things!!

This can be a very powerful concept to teach children.

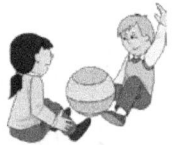

By helping them understand this early on –

We can then go on to teach them healthier

ways of coping with their feelings!

Another way I like to ask people look at **EMOTIONS:**

Have you ever said things you wished you hadn't?

Here's WHY it happens:

Feelings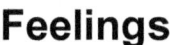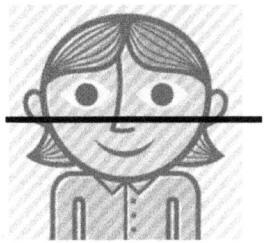

When feelings build up to here -
You have *NO CONTROL* over what comes out!

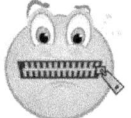 At this level it is best
NOT TO
OPEN YOUR MOUTH!

These are the words you can't take back!

There is *one more level!*

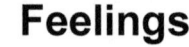 **Feelings**

"I can't believe I DID THAT!"

This is when feelings build up so high
the brain gets **flooded** & can't think straight!

This also happens to other people & is why

I teach it is BEST to

WAIT to talk with someone!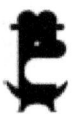

If their emotions are **that high,**

They **WON'T** be able to

HEAR what's being said:

The **FEELINGS** are 'covering up their 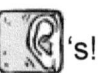's!

So, hopefully you can begin to

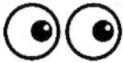

what is going on with our EMOTIONS.

It is only when we *start* to be AWARE

that we can *start* to **have success!**

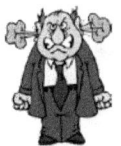
This brings us to

the next step:

Managing Emotions

Now that we understand how emotions

can manage us -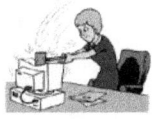

It's time to look at

WHAT we can do to manage them.

Don't worry – it's simpler than you think!

Managing Emotions

2 Steps to Success:

Step 1 - STOP the level from rising!

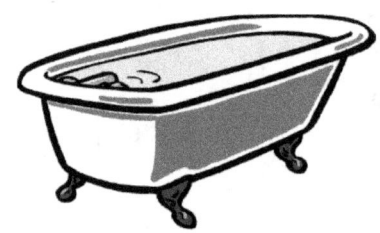

If we don't do something to

    STOP the level from rising –

        it will ....OVERFLOW!

Leaving a BIG MESS to clean up!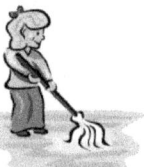

These actions will be PASSIVE –

meaning they don't require much energy!

Step 2 - **RELEASE** so the level drops!

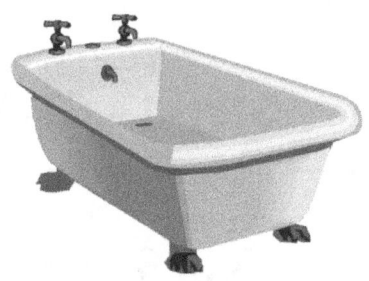

The only way to get rid of what's there is…..

to let it out!

These actions must be *ACTIVE* –

muscle involvement must be used!

The MISTAKE people make ➡ only do 1 step!

This DOESN"T work!

Imagine the tub above…….

So let's say we only **STOP** *the level from rising.*

What happens a bit later when it starts to rise again?

A BIG MESS to clean up!!!

You can see –

The same principle applies to the bottles!

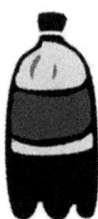

Step 1 - STOP
the pressure from building

Step 2 - RELEASE
the pressure that's there!

Once again, If we only do **Step 1** -

the pressure in the bottle remains there!

Most likely to come out on the WRONG person...

That's what used to happen to me!

During a really difficult day at work, I'd
find myself feeling frustrated & annoyed.

Listening to music helped me calm down....

The problem was if something else **at home**
annoyed or frustrated me – *I'd lose it!*

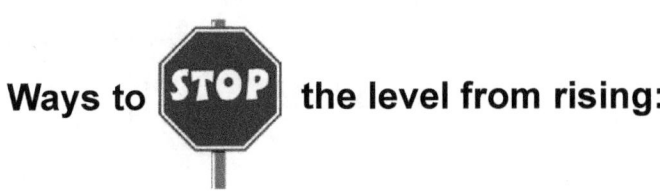 **Ways to STOP the level from rising:**

Reading

Breathing

Count to 10

Listen to music

Meditation

Prayer

Time out

Guided imagery

Thought stopping

+ self-talk

Change your environment

More →

More ways to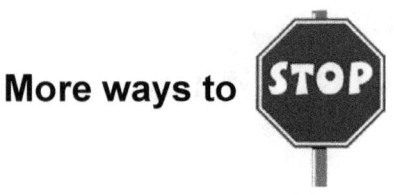

Serenity Prayer

Mental Foxhole

Reframing:

- Don't take it personal

- It is what it is

Let go

Hot shower or bath

Looking at a picture

Aromatherapy

Self-care

Maybe you have some others you can think of -

Any "calming" activity will work here!

Ways to 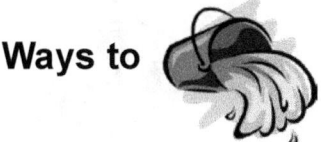 what's there

Talk

Write

Scream in the car

Punching bag

Clean

Sing / Dance

Exercise / Walk

Constructive destruction

Pace

Air box

Laugh

More →

More ways to

Climb some stairs

Cry

Push up / Sit ups

Call someone

Tear up phone book

Split wood

Gardening

Empty chair method

Cooking

Mow the lawn

Wash the car

**Any activity requiring muscle involvement

Important:

Before going on to Step 2 – RELEASE

You must **make sure** you have done Step 1.

DO NOT SKIP STEP 1!

This system will not work if you haven't stopped the feelings from building up!

In fact,

You will end up with the opposite:

A BIGGER MESS of emotion.

It's very similar to what happens when we have a fire already going & we throw gasoline on it!

It GETS BIGGER!

One other point I would like to make –

There is…..

no one size that fits all

The ideas I've listed on the previous pages

will not work the same for everyone.

You job is to try out different ones

& see which one will work best for you!

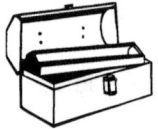
Be sure to get a good variety in your toolbox.

After all, those of us wearing glasses

Have a couple different size screwdrivers!

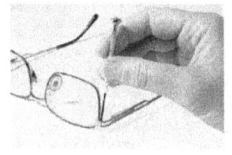 ➕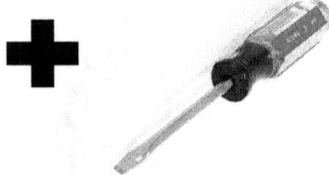

You can never have *too many* tools!

To keep things SIMPLE

the following can be helpful!

"The Quick 3!"

Walk **Talk** **Write / Dump**

Dumping is when you write,

However, you don't read

what you just wrote!

Instead, you DESTROY IT!

This is different from "Journaling".

With Dumping –

The goal is to just get it **out of your brain!**

When you **read** it – it **reloads** it!

It would be like taking a bucket
and dumping water out of the boat,

Then scooping up water & putting back in the boat!

** "Dumping" also works really well when you can't fall asleep because your mind is racing or if you wake up & your mind is racing!

For fun - you can even make a "Dump Box"!

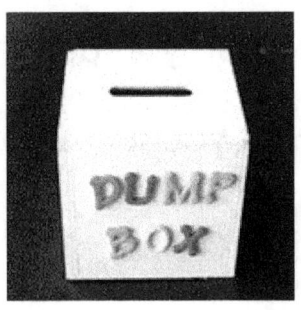

A few more Wordtools

to help get the point across:

Definitely

Why

Emotions

Last

Longer!

© 2017 & licensed by Well YOUniversity, LLC
Taken from "Words at Work"

BE CAREFUL!!!

This is what many people are good at doing!

When we are using LifeTOOLS

instead of Survival Tools

this is what we are doing!

Accessing

Coping

Tools

© 2017 & licensed by Well YOUniversity, LLC
Taken from "Words at Work"

When we are using Survival Tools

& NOT USING LifeTOOLS

This is what we do:

Release

Emotion

And

Create

Trouble!

© 2017 & licensed by Well YOUniversity, LLC
Taken from "Words at Work"

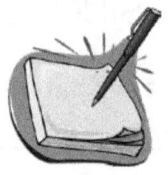

Sign up now!

To get access to updates, more tools, coaching calls, and upcoming events

Text: SELFNESS

To: **44222**

Another exercise I like to do in my live events –

Is to see how many cars people have owned!

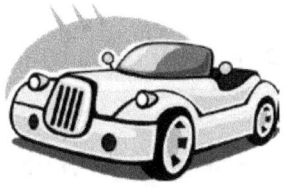

I'll ask people to raise their hands -

1

3

5*

(This includes new, used, hand-me-downs, & ones that don't run anymore!)

How about you? What number? _____

If you've NEVER owned a car – I got you covered!
I'll explain on the next page!

***** I stop here – Don't want to give anyone's age away!

Now Imagine….

You had 1 car that had to last you a lifetime.

How well would you take care of that car?!

If you're like the folks in my events, you answered:

Pretty Darn Well!

So, here's what I want you to understand –

You're reading this book in the '**one car**" you own!

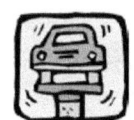
It's called your BODY

&

It has to last you a lifetime…

So how are you doing?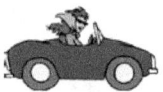

Are you taking really good care of your **"Life Car"**?

The secret to keeping your **one car** running?

Self-Care!

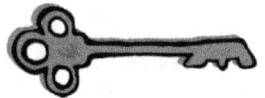

#3

Have a
Solid Foundation

When I ask this question in a live event every hand in the room goes up!

"How many of you already KNOW that in order to be well you need to?"

Exercise

Have good nutrition

Manage stress

Follow up w/ medical stuff?

Again, that's SMARTheory at work!

So what we will cover next probably

won't be  information"

Instead,

I am going to help you 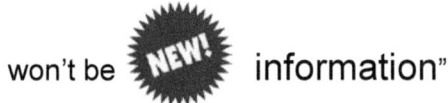 those things *a little differently!*

I'd like to introduce you to the:

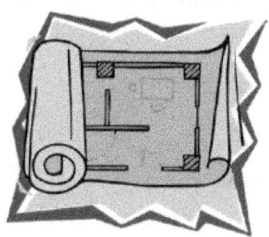

L.I.F.E Wellness Blueprint

I created this blueprint 25 years ago!

It is what I've used to stay well since then

&

what I have taught to **1,000's**

in the hospital programs where I've worked!

Blueprints are amazing!

If you follow them – you end up with the same thing EVERY TIME!!!

Before we go any further -

I want to share with you my favorite Wordtool

Living

Intentionally &

Fully

Engaged!

© 2017 & licensed by Well YOUniversity, LLC
Taken from "Words at Work"

I need you to imagine…

I'm standing on a 4-legged chair right in front of you!

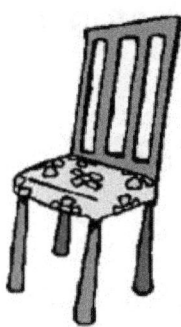

You saw off one of the legs….

What do you think will happen? Do I fall on you?!

Probably not –

since I have 3 legs I can still shift my weight to!

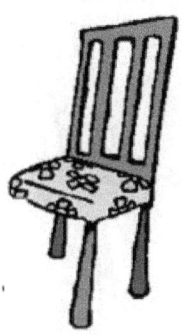

After all,

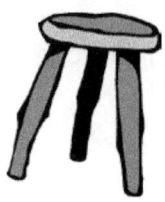 A stool only has 3 legs!

I'll bet you have probably sat on one of these!

The problem with stools is they aren't too sturdy!

I have sat on a 3-legged stool

AND I have tipped over on one….

You come along & saw off another leg!

What happens to me now?!

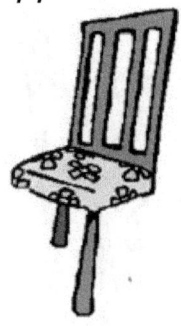

The truth is …….

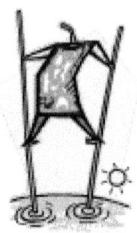

I could only stay up on those things for a short time!

Even if I was good at stilts -

it wouldn't take *much of a bump to knock me over.*

(We all know **LIFE IS FULL OF BUMPS**!).

Now, you saw off the 3rd leg -

                        Leaving me with only 1!!!!

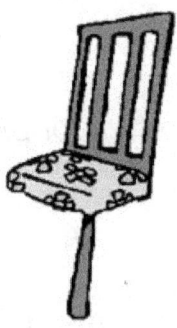

What do you think is going to happen to me?

You're right!   ***I'm going down…***

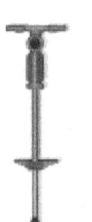

Oops!

I never could pogo stick!

So, when we expect just

Exercise or nutrition

to keep us going…..

IT CAN"T – IT IS ONLY 1 LEG!

Self Care

(Pretty wobbly!)

As you can see, this is what

the blueprint would

look like with just that…..

Building a STRONG Foundation!

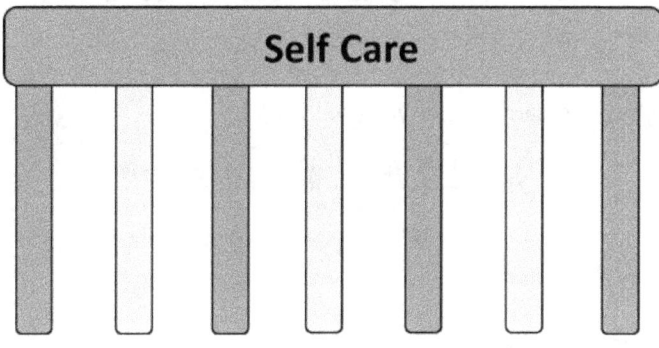

(MUCH better!)

This is what a complete blueprint of the foundation looks like!

Now, I want you to imagine me standing on this chair with **7** legs...

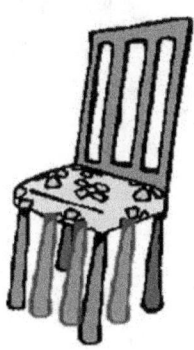

Don't you agree that would give us a
"**solid**, "**strong**", "**stable**", "**sturdy**" foundation?!!

This is exactly how you will find
your *L.I.F.E. foundation*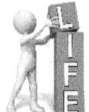
When you build out this blueprint!

The reason we need to have such a solid foundation is because of this *thing* called STRESS!

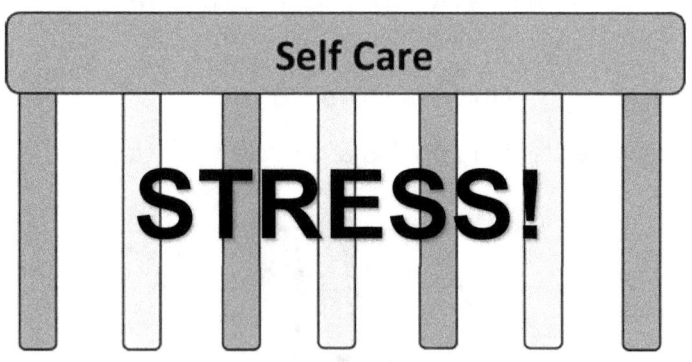

I like to teach that
STRESS is *like an earthquake*!

It can really shake up our lives!

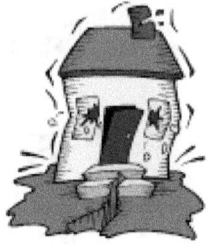

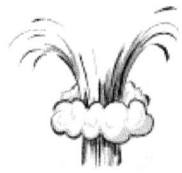　Foundations tend to take a bruising during earthquakes & parts have been known to fall down.

We've got to make sure

WE HAVE PLENTY of foundation!

When we **START** to *lose some of it*

to **BIG STRESS** going on in our lives

or

a **WHOLE BUNCH** of little stresses -

We've got to have enough left to keep us **standing!**

Lost some!

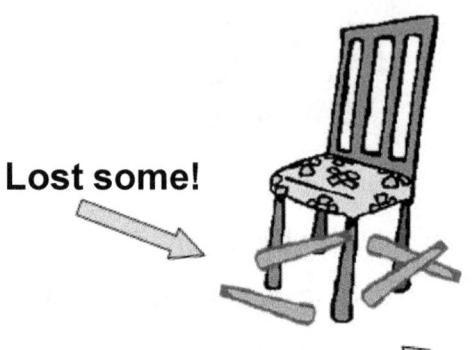

Still have some left!

It could even be that

the **STRESS** of caregiving

has *taken down* what you had in place

as your **existing foundation**

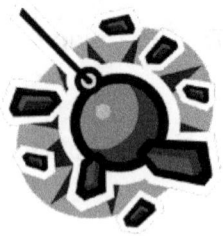

The Foundation Corners!

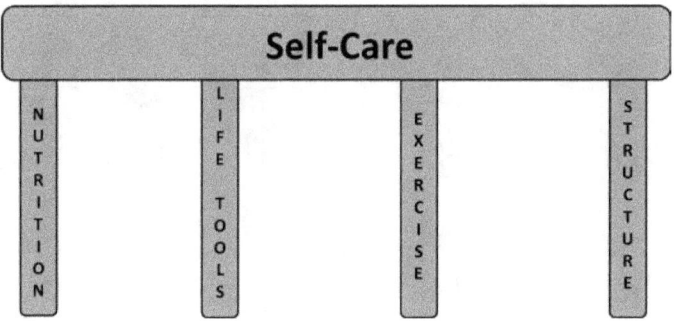

This is *how* the things we KNOW we NEED to do

Nutrition

    Exercise

        Life Tools

            Structure

FIT TOGETHER!

Can you SEE why we can't just rely

on exercise or nutrition alone....

It only works when

ALL 4 Foundation Corners are there!

The BIG Picture!

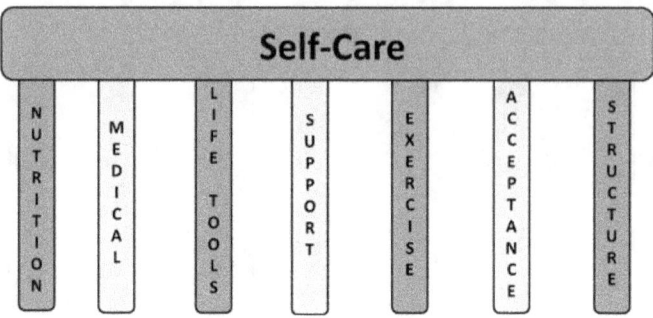

Now when we ADD the others –

Medical ➡ Keep current on medical stuff!

Support ➡ Have **+** people around us!

Acceptance ➡ KNOW you *need* to do this!

We have an even

STRONGER FOUNDATION OF

Self-Care!

I have two stories I'd like to share to help understand how this applies to you!

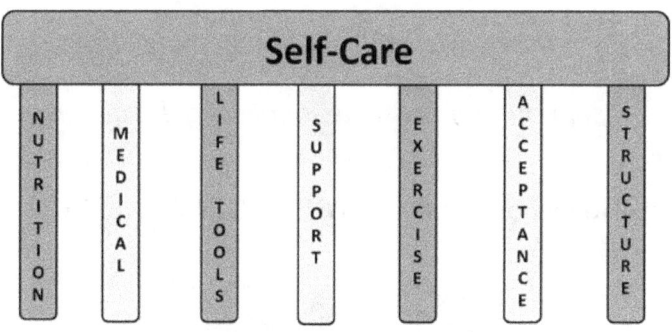

This is Peter's foundation.

He lives with a chronic health issue – diabetes & has been *doing well* for the past **5 years.**

He suddenly found himself becoming **the primary caregiver** for his elderly parents.

This meant every day he had to drive **45** miles one-way to get to their house.

Things went OK to start, then they started needing more help, Peter's life was turned upside down……

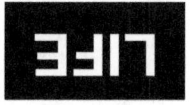

So he lost his **STRUCTURE:**

His routine had been a solid one:

going to the gym, healthy meals, go to his diabetes support group, & time for playing the guitar!

He lost one of his **FOUNDATION CORNERS.**

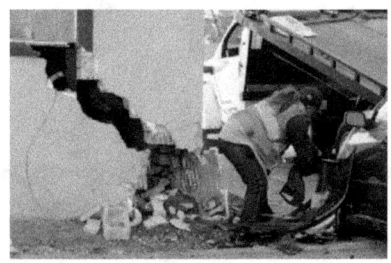

That's like losing one corner of your house!

His Self-Care Blueprint took a hit & became this:

Self-Care					
NUTRITION	MEDICAL	LIFE TOOLS	SUPPORT	EXERCISE	ACCEPTANCE

As he needed to spend more time at his parents, he lost another FOUNDATION CORNER: EXERCISE

So now his Self –Care looked like this:

Self-Care

| NUTRITION | MEDICAL | LIFE TOOLS | SUPPORT | ACCEPTANCE |

When we lose one of the **4** foundation corners it sets off a '***domino effect***' & others start to fall.

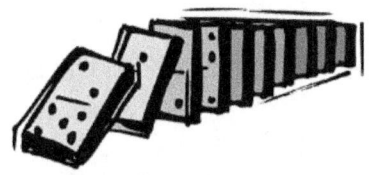

In Peter's case, it happened pretty quickly.

Within just a couple months his diabetes

was out of control………

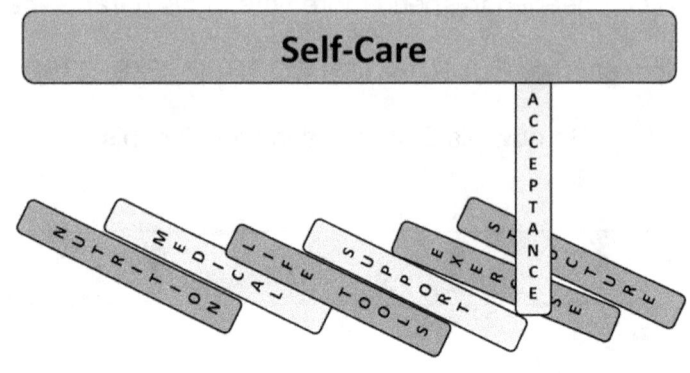

Here's what Peter's foundation looked like.

This is ***not enough***

to keep ANYONE healthy & well!

Without his foundation…….. Peter ended up

Self-Care

HOSPITALIZED

The chronic illness he lived with took over.

Now I'd like to tell you Mary's story.

Self-Care

| NUTRITION | MEDICAL | LIFE TOOLS | SUPPORT | EXERCISE | ACCEPTANCE | STRUCTURE |

This is Mary's foundation.

She **has no chronic health issues.**

In fact, she's in the **best health** of her life!

Mary started a new job as a case manager.

She'd studied social work in school & was excited!

After 6 months, Mary was putting in a lot of hours.

Too exhausted once she got home, she started missing days at her gym.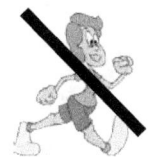

She did some walking every day at lunchtime –

but this was limited to only **5-10** minutes.

So she lost her **EXERCISE:**

Her routine had been a solid one:

She'd go to the gym 6 days a week. Her workout included strength training, cardio exercise, & yoga!

She lost one of her **FOUNDATION CORNERS.**

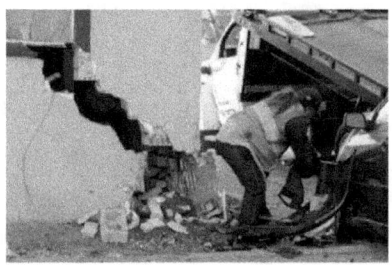

That's like losing one corner of your house!

Her Self-Care blueprint took a hit & became this:

Self-Care						
NUTRITION	MEDICAL	LIFE TOOLS	SUPPORT		ACCEPTANCE	STRUCTURE

As she continued to work *A LOT HOURS*
& her schedule remained very hectic

She lost another 1 ½ FOUNDATION CORNERS::

LIFETOOLS & ½ NUTRITION

So now her Self –Care looked like this:

Self-Care

| NUTRITION | MEDICAL | SUPPORT | | ACCEPTANCE | STRUCTURE |

Remember the dominoes!

Lose one of the **4** foundation corners

it sets off a ***chain reaction*** & others start to fall.

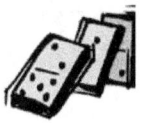
In Mary's case, stress & work demands took its toll on her health. She stopped most of her SELF-CARE.

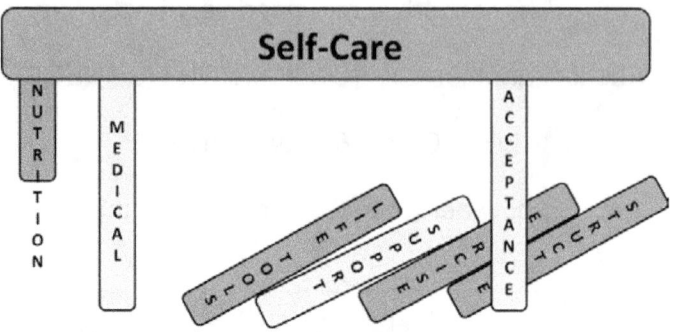

Here's what Mary's foundation looked like.

This was **not enough**

to keep ANYONE healthy & well!

With a limited foundation…….. Mary ended up

Self-Care

IN TREATMENT FOR MIGRAINES

She developed a chronic health issue.

Wrapping Up

What We've Covered

We started out introducing you to

 SELFNESS!

NO, you **aren't being SELFISH** when

you takes steps to care for yourself 1st.

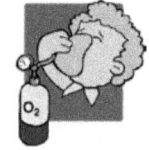

Remember:

If you don't put the oxygen mask on yourself 1st

You won't be able to help

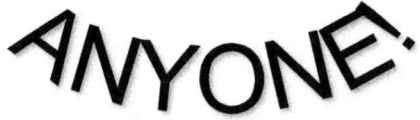

Don't let somebody tell you otherwise!

Then we went on to

3 Keys of Self-Care Success!

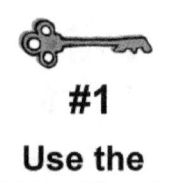

#1

**Use the
*Right Tools!***

The 1st thing to do:

Check & see if you are using any old

SURVIVAL TOOLS.

These may have served you
well in the past… (They got you to here!)

However, ***moving forward*** they
can become The BIGGER Problem.

The 2nd thing to do: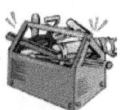

Make sure you have a **FULL TOOLBOX!**

There is no 'one tool fixes all.'

You can never have too many **LifeTOOLS!**

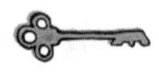

#2
Manage Your Emotions!

Although it may **not SEEM like it**

FEELINGS & BEHAVIORS

Are 2 *Different* things!

FEELING	BEHAVIOR
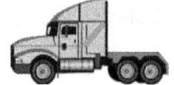	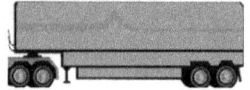

We are responsible to CHOOSE!

Remember,

The Secret to Success is

picking a NEW behavior you can **DO** immediately!

Walk   **Talk**   **Write / Dump**

Then there's **WHAT** we can do to

Managing Emotions

2 Steps to Success:

Step 1 - STOP the level from rising!

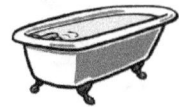

Step 2 – RELEASE so the level drops!

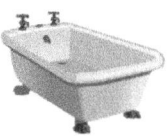

Lastly………

When the feelings build up to this level

Feelings 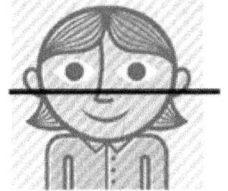   *DO NOT* **OPEN YOUR MOUTH!**

Otherwise you will say things you can't take back.

#3
Have a *Solid* Foundation

This is the last key we looked at!

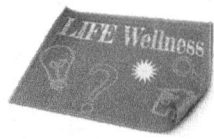

There is no doubt you will experience some

STRESS in your life........

It all comes down to: How strong of

a foundation do you have?

THIS

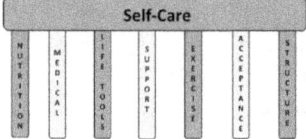

or

THAT

Self-Care
HOSPITALIZED

A Quick Check-Out!

So I said this would be again at the end! Circle the number below each statement that best describes where you are RIGHT NOW!

1) I feel I have enough self-care tools.

    0   1   2   3   4   5

not at all!   absolutely

2) I use self-care tools every day.

    0   1   2   3   4   5

not at all!   absolutely

3) I feel I have a right to take time for myself.

    0   1   2   3   4   5

not at all!   absolutely

BONUS:

Send me an email with before & after scores! I'll give you a 30-minute coaching call with me!!!

Carol@WellYOUniversity.com   Subject: Selfness

Limited number of slots available!

We'd love to hear from you!

Feedback Card

Please take a moment & provide us some feedback about the book you just read & how you feel *it benefited YOU!*

_____

_____

_____

_____

Tear along here

Name: _____

Best Phone #: _____

Can we use your comments in our publicity materials?
Yes / No

If OK with you, what's the best time to call you:_____

Thank You!

Scan or take a picture & email:
      Carol@WellYOUniversity.com

Snail mail: Carol Rickard
    5 Zion Rd, Hopewell, NJ 08525

About the Author

Carol L Rickard, LCSW, TTS, of Hopewell, NJ is founder & CEO of WellYOUniversity, LLC, a global health education company dedicated *to empowering individuals with the tools and supports to achieve lifelong wellness & recovery.*

Also known as **America's Wellness Ambassador**, Carol is a dynamic & engaging speaker who brings to life practical / useful solutions. She is a weekly contributor for Esperanza Magazine; written 13 books on stress and wellness, had a guest appearance on Dr. Oz this past winter.

She is also the creator & host of a 30-minute wellness show on Princeton TV - **The WELL YOU Show** which can be seen at:

www.vimeo.com/channels/wellyou

Get more of Carol at:

Twitter: ***@wellYOUlife***

"Like us" @ www.FaceBook.com/WellYOUniversity

Have Carol Speak at Your Next Event!

Get more information about how you can have Carol speak at your organization, event, or conference.

Go to: www.CarolLRickard.com

Or call: 888 Life Tools (543-3866)

Carol's Other Books

Stress Eating

Stretched Not Broken

The Caregiver's Toolbox

Transforming Illness to Wellness

Putting Your Weight Loss on Auto

The Benefits of Smoking

Moving Beyond Depression

LifeTools

Words At Work Vol. 1

Words at Work Vol. 2

Creating Compliance

Relapse Prevention

Please visit us at:

www.WellYOUniversity.com

Sign up for weekly motivational e-quote!

Check out our upcoming FREE webinars!

Learn more about our training programs.

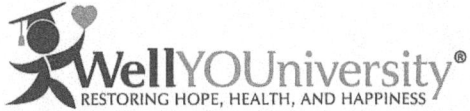

Email us your success story at:

Success@WellYOUniversity.com

We'd like to ask for your feedback

Please check out the last page
if this book has been HELPFUL for you!

www.ingramcontent.com/pod-product-compliance
Lightning Source LLC
LaVergne TN
LVHW051842080426
835512LV00018B/3021